THE COMPLETE

DR BARBARA

CURE FOR

ERECTILE

DYSFUNCTION

A DETAILED GUIDE TO REVERSE ERECTILE
DYSFUNCTION WITH DR. BARBARA O'NEILL
INSPIRED NATURAL HERBAL REMEDIES

Ellis Moss

TABLE OF CONTENTS

INTRODUCTION

In the realm of men's health, erectile dysfunction (ED) has long been a shrouded topic, often associated with shame and embarrassment. Yet, it's a prevalent condition that affects millions worldwide. For those struggling with ED, the search for effective solutions can be a daunting journey.

Enter Dr. Barbara, a renowned expert in the field of men's health and sexual dysfunction. With years of dedicated research and clinical experience, Dr. Barbara has pioneered innovative approaches to address ED. Her ground-breaking work has transformed the way we understand and treat this condition.

The complete Dr. Barbara's Cure for Erectile Dysfunction offers a comprehensive guide to understanding and overcoming ED. This book is a beacon of hope for men seeking to regain their confidence, intimacy, and overall well-being.

Throughout the pages of this book Dr. Barbara inspired book the author delves into the root causes of ED, exploring both physical and psychological factors that can contribute to this condition. She provides clear explanations of the latest medical advancements and treatment options, empowering readers to make informed decisions about their healthcare.

Beyond medical interventions, Dr. Barbara emphasizes the importance of lifestyle factors in maintaining sexual health. She offers practical advice on diet, exercise, stress management, and relationship dynamics, providing a holistic approach to addressing ED.

Whether you are seeking information, support, or a path to recovery, *Dr. Barbara's Cure for Erectile*

Dysfunction is an invaluable resource. This book empowers men to take control of their health, reclaim their sexual vitality, and embark on a journey toward a more fulfilling and satisfying life.

UNDERSTANDING ERECTILE DYSFUNCTION

Erectile dysfunction, simply put, is the inability to achieve or maintain an erection that is firm enough for sexual intercourse. It's a complex issue with a variety of underlying causes, including physical, psychological, and lifestyle factors. While it can be a sensitive topic to discuss, it's important to remember that ED is a common health problem and that seeking help is a sign of strength, not weakness.

Recognizing the Signs

If you're experiencing difficulties with erections, it's essential to pay attention to the signs and symptoms. Some common indicators of ED include:

- **Difficulty achieving or maintaining an erection:** This is the most obvious symptom, but it can manifest in different ways.
- **Decreased sexual desire:** A loss of interest in sex can sometimes be a precursor to ED.
- **Premature ejaculation:** If you find yourself ejaculating too quickly, it might be a sign of underlying erectile dysfunction.
- **Painful erections:** Discomfort or pain during or after sex can be a cause for concern.

Why This Book Matters

Dr. Barbara's book offers a beacon of hope for men struggling with ED. Through her years of experience and research, she has developed a holistic approach to addressing this condition. This guide will provide you with:

- **Comprehensive information:** Learn about the causes, symptoms, and treatment options for ED.
- **Practical advice:** Discover lifestyle changes, dietary recommendations, and exercises that can improve erectile function.
- **Support and guidance:** Understand the psychological impact of ED and find strategies to boost your confidence and self-esteem.
- **Personalized solutions:** Explore a variety of treatment options, including medications, therapy, and medical devices.

Are you ready to take control of your sexual health and rediscover your vitality? Join us on this journey as we delve into the world of erectile dysfunction and explore the groundbreaking solutions offered by Dr. Barbara.

DR BARBARA FOR ERECTILE DYSFUNCTION

Dr. Barbara O'Neill is a well-known health practitioner and naturopath who advocates for natural healing methods through lifestyle changes, diet, and holistic remedies. Her approach is based on the idea that many diseases and conditions can be prevented or managed by addressing the underlying causes, rather than just treating symptoms with pharmaceuticals. When it comes to erectile dysfunction (ED), her philosophy aligns with the concept of healing the body from within, using natural, non-invasive strategies that target the root causes of this condition.

Understanding Erectile Dysfunction (ED)

Erectile dysfunction is the inability to achieve or maintain an erection sufficient for sexual intercourse. It affects millions of men globally and can lead to psychological stress, relationship issues, and reduced self-esteem. While occasional ED is normal and can be caused by temporary factors such as stress or fatigue, chronic ED is usually a sign of an underlying health problem, which could be linked to cardiovascular diseases, diabetes, hormonal imbalances, or mental health disorders.

Conventional treatments for ED include medications such as phosphodiesterase inhibitors (like Viagra and Cialis), hormone therapy, or mechanical devices. While these treatments may provide temporary relief, they often do not address the root causes of the problem, and long-term dependence on medication may have side effects.

Dr. Barbara O'Neill's approach to erectile dysfunction would center around addressing lifestyle factors that could be contributing to the condition. She believes in using natural remedies, detoxification, and dietary changes to restore the body's natural balance. Here are several key areas that Dr. Barbara would focus on when dealing with ED:

1. Diet and Nutrition

Diet plays a significant role in managing erectile dysfunction. Poor circulation, inflammation, and hormone imbalances are often linked to dietary habits. Dr. Barbara advocates for a plant-based, anti-inflammatory diet that includes:

- **Whole foods**: Fresh fruits and vegetables that are rich in antioxidants can improve blood flow and reduce inflammation.

- **Healthy fats**: Omega-3 fatty acids found in fish, flaxseeds, and walnuts can help improve circulation and reduce inflammation, which are crucial for combating ED.
- **Elimination of processed foods and sugar**: Processed foods, refined sugars, and unhealthy fats can cause insulin resistance, contribute to weight gain, and lead to diabetes—all risk factors for ED.
- **Increased intake of zinc and magnesium**: Zinc is essential for testosterone production, and magnesium helps relax blood vessels, improving circulation.

Dr. Barbara might also encourage specific foods known to enhance sexual health, such as watermelon, which contains citrulline that improves blood flow, or dark leafy greens like spinach, which are high in nitric oxide.

2. Detoxification and Gut Health

Dr. Barbara O'Neill often emphasizes the importance of detoxifying the body to eliminate toxins that may hinder its natural healing processes. She believes that a healthy gut is the foundation of good health, including sexual health. A compromised gut can lead to inflammation, hormone imbalances, and poor absorption of nutrients, all of which can contribute to ED.

Her detox methods might include:

- **Juicing**: A regular juicing regimen with ingredients like leafy greens, beets, and carrots can help cleanse the liver and improve circulation. A healthy liver is essential for hormone balance, which directly impacts sexual function.

- **Fasting and cleansing**: Periodic fasting or detox protocols can help the body eliminate toxins and reset hormonal balance.

Improving gut health with fermented foods like sauerkraut, kimchi, and kefir would also be part of her strategy. Probiotics could play a role in improving the gut flora, which helps with nutrient absorption and inflammation reduction.

3. Managing Stress and Mental Health

Stress, anxiety, and depression are major contributors to erectile dysfunction. Dr. Barbara would likely emphasize the importance of managing stress through natural methods. Chronic stress increases the production of cortisol, a hormone that can interfere with testosterone production, which is critical for male sexual health.

Her recommendations might include:

- **Regular physical activity**: Exercise, particularly strength training and cardiovascular activities, not only improves circulation but also reduces stress and boosts testosterone levels.

- **Relaxation techniques**: Meditation, deep-breathing exercises, and yoga can help manage stress and improve overall mental health.

- **Sleep hygiene**: Lack of sleep disrupts hormone balance, particularly testosterone production, and contributes to stress and fatigue. Dr. Barbara would likely suggest improving sleep quality through natural methods like avoiding stimulants, creating a bedtime routine, and reducing exposure to electronic screens before bed.

4. Improving Circulation and Cardiovascular Health

ED is often linked to poor blood flow and cardiovascular issues. Dr. Barbara would address this by promoting practices that naturally improve circulation and heart health.

- **Exercise**: Regular aerobic exercise, such as walking, running, or swimming, improves circulation and strengthens the heart, which is vital for erectile function.
- **Herbal remedies**: Dr. Barbara might recommend herbs such as **ginkgo biloba**, which is known to enhance blood flow, or **maca root**, which is believed to boost libido and energy levels.
- **Hydration**: Proper hydration is critical for blood flow. Dehydration can cause blood vessels to constrict, limiting circulation and exacerbating ED symptoms.

5. Hormonal Balance

Hormone imbalances, particularly low testosterone, are a significant cause of erectile dysfunction. Dr. Barbara's natural approach to restoring hormonal balance would involve:

- **Dietary changes**: Foods rich in zinc, magnesium, and vitamin D would be prioritized, as they play a critical role in hormone production and regulation.

- **Reducing exposure to endocrine disruptors**: Chemicals found in plastics, pesticides, and personal care products can mimic or block hormones in the body, leading to imbalances. Dr. Barbara would advocate for reducing exposure to these chemicals by using natural, non-toxic products.

- **Herbal supplements**: Adaptogenic herbs such as **ashwagandha** and **rhodiola** can help balance hormones by reducing stress and supporting the endocrine system.

Dr. Barbara O'Neill's approach to erectile dysfunction is rooted in holistic wellness, focusing on healing the body from within rather than relying on medications that mask symptoms. By addressing diet, detoxification, stress, circulation, and hormonal balance, her methods aim to target the root causes of ED. For men dealing with erectile dysfunction, this natural approach offers a comprehensive way to not only improve sexual function but also enhance overall health and well-being.

THE ROLE OF NUTRITION IN ERECTILE DYSFUNCTION

Erectile dysfunction (ED) is a condition where a man is unable to achieve or maintain an erection sufficient for sexual intercourse. It can have various causes, including psychological, hormonal, or physical factors. One of the most crucial but often overlooked factors in managing and preventing ED is nutrition. The foods we consume play a fundamental role in almost every aspect of health, including sexual health. Good nutrition can help prevent or alleviate ED by promoting better blood flow, balancing hormones, and supporting overall cardiovascular health, while poor dietary choices can exacerbate the problem.

How Nutrition Affects Erectile Dysfunction

1. Blood Flow and Circulation

For an erection to occur, adequate blood flow to the penis is essential. Nutrients that promote healthy circulation help maintain the integrity of blood vessels and ensure smooth blood flow. Foods rich in antioxidants, nitrates, and certain vitamins can improve circulation and help prevent the narrowing and hardening of arteries (atherosclerosis), a key contributor to ED.

- **Antioxidants**: These protect the blood vessels from oxidative stress, a form of cellular damage that can lead to impaired blood flow. Fruits and vegetables, especially berries, citrus fruits, and leafy greens, are excellent sources of antioxidants.

- **Nitrates**: Found in vegetables like spinach, beets, and arugula, nitrates help dilate blood vessels, improving circulation. This vasodilation effect directly impacts erectile function by allowing for better blood flow to the penis.

2. Testosterone Production and Hormonal Balance

Testosterone is the primary male hormone responsible for libido, energy, and overall sexual function. Nutritional deficiencies can disrupt testosterone production, leading to low libido and poor sexual performance. A diet rich in zinc, magnesium, vitamin D, and healthy fats is essential for maintaining normal testosterone levels.

- **Zinc**: This mineral is necessary for testosterone production and overall sexual health. Oysters, red meat, pumpkin seeds, and legumes are rich sources of zinc. A deficiency in zinc can lead to reduced testosterone levels and poor sperm quality, directly impacting erectile function.

- **Vitamin D**: Low levels of vitamin D are associated with erectile dysfunction and decreased testosterone production. Sun exposure, fortified foods, and fatty fish like salmon are excellent ways to boost vitamin D levels.

3. Obesity and Weight Management

Obesity is a significant risk factor for erectile dysfunction. Excess body fat can lead to hormonal imbalances (such as increased estrogen and lower testosterone levels), insulin resistance, and inflammation—all of which contribute to ED. Poor diet choices, especially those high in processed foods, refined sugars, and unhealthy fats, promote weight gain and obesity, further compounding the risk.

- **Insulin Resistance**: A diet high in refined carbohydrates and sugars leads to insulin resistance, a precursor to type 2 diabetes, which is closely linked to erectile dysfunction. Diabetes can cause nerve damage (neuropathy) and poor blood circulation, both of which affect sexual function.
- **Inflammation**: A diet high in unhealthy fats, such as trans fats, can trigger chronic inflammation, which damages blood vessels and impairs blood flow, increasing the risk of ED.

Certain foods are especially beneficial for improving sexual health and preventing erectile dysfunction. These foods promote better circulation, boost testosterone levels, reduce inflammation, and support overall health.

1. Leafy Green Vegetables

Vegetables like spinach, kale, and arugula are rich in nitrates, which help improve blood flow by promoting the dilation of blood vessels. Nitric oxide, a compound produced in the body from nitrates, is essential for maintaining an erection. Nitric oxide relaxes the smooth muscles of blood vessels, allowing blood to flow more freely to the penis.

2. Berries and Citrus Fruits

Berries such as blueberries, strawberries, and blackberries are loaded with antioxidants, particularly flavonoids, which help protect blood vessels from oxidative damage. Studies show that men who consume higher amounts of flavonoids from fruits are less likely to develop ED. Citrus fruits, including oranges, lemons, and grapefruits, also contain flavonoids that enhance circulation and reduce the risk of ED.

3. Nuts and Seeds

Nuts like almonds, walnuts, and Brazil nuts are rich in essential fatty acids, particularly omega-3s, which support heart health and circulation. Brazil nuts are a particularly good source of selenium, a mineral that plays a role in hormone production and sexual function. Pumpkin seeds are high in zinc, crucial for testosterone production and overall sexual health.

4. Oysters and Shellfish

Oysters are famously known as an aphrodisiac due to their high zinc content, a mineral crucial for testosterone production. Shellfish, in general, provides a good source of zinc, which helps maintain healthy hormone levels and boosts libido.

5. Fatty Fish

Fish like salmon, mackerel, and sardines are rich in omega-3 fatty acids, which help reduce inflammation and improve cardiovascular health. Omega-3s promote better blood flow and protect the lining of blood vessels, reducing the risk of ED. Fatty fish is also an excellent source of vitamin D, which is linked to improved testosterone levels.

6. Dark Chocolate

Dark chocolate, particularly varieties that contain at least 70% cocoa, is a rich source of flavonoids, which help improve circulation by promoting nitric oxide production. The antioxidants in dark chocolate also help reduce blood pressure and inflammation, further benefiting erectile function.

7. Watermelon

Watermelon contains an amino acid called citrulline, which helps to increase the production of nitric oxide. This can improve blood flow to the penis and potentially help with mild cases of ED. Watermelon is often referred to as "nature's Viagra" because of its ability to enhance blood flow similarly to how ED medications work.

8. Garlic and Onions

Garlic and onions are known for their heart-healthy benefits. They help thin the blood and promote better circulation by preventing the formation of clots. Better blood flow is essential for achieving and maintaining an erection, so including these in your diet can have a positive impact on sexual health.

9. Pomegranate

Pomegranate juice is rich in antioxidants, particularly polyphenols, which help to improve blood circulation. Studies have shown that pomegranate juice may help improve erectile function in men by reducing oxidative stress and enhancing blood flow.

10. Tomatoes

Tomatoes are rich in lycopene, a powerful antioxidant that helps improve circulation and protect against cardiovascular disease. Studies suggest that lycopene may help improve sperm quality and reduce the risk of prostate cancer, indirectly supporting better sexual health.

Nutritional Deficiencies and Their Impact on Erectile Dysfunction

Nutritional deficiencies can have a profound impact on erectile function. Deficiencies in certain vitamins and minerals can lead to hormonal imbalances, poor circulation, and reduced sexual performance. Here are some common deficiencies linked to ED and their effects:

1. Zinc Deficiency

Zinc is essential for testosterone production and maintaining healthy sexual function. A deficiency in zinc can lead to reduced testosterone levels, decreased libido, and poor sperm quality. Men who are deficient in zinc may experience erectile difficulties due to lower testosterone levels.

2. Vitamin D Deficiency

Vitamin D is crucial for maintaining testosterone levels. Low vitamin D is associated with reduced nitric oxide production and impaired blood flow, which can contribute to erectile dysfunction. Additionally, a lack of vitamin D can increase the risk of cardiovascular problems, further exacerbating ED symptoms.

3. Magnesium Deficiency

Magnesium plays a role in relaxing blood vessels and supporting proper blood flow. A deficiency in magnesium can lead to elevated blood pressure, which can impair circulation and contribute to ED. Magnesium also helps regulate testosterone levels, so low magnesium can impact sexual performance.

4. B Vitamin Deficiency

B vitamins, particularly B12 and folate, are essential for nerve function and blood flow. Deficiencies in these vitamins can cause nerve damage, which may impair the signals required for an erection. Additionally, B vitamins support cardiovascular health, and a deficiency can increase the risk of cardiovascular diseases linked to ED.

5. Omega-3 Fatty Acid Deficiency

Omega-3s are important for heart health and reducing inflammation. A diet low in omega-3s can lead to increased inflammation, poor circulation, and an elevated risk of cardiovascular diseases—all of which contribute to ED. Omega-3 fatty acids are also known to improve endothelial function, which is critical for maintaining healthy blood flow.

THE ROLE OF HERBAL MEDICINE IN TREATING ERECTILE DYSFUNCTION (ED)

Herbal medicine has been used for centuries to treat a wide range of health issues, including sexual health concerns like erectile dysfunction (ED). While modern pharmaceuticals such as Viagra and Cialis have become common treatments for ED, many men seek natural alternatives due to concerns over side effects, dependency, or a desire for more holistic health approaches. Herbal medicine offers a variety of natural remedies that have shown promising effects in managing ED by improving blood flow, enhancing libido, balancing hormones, and reducing stress.

How Herbal Medicine Affects and Helps Erectile Dysfunction Patients

Erectile dysfunction often has complex underlying causes, including poor circulation, stress, hormonal imbalances, or psychological issues like anxiety and depression. Herbal remedies work by addressing these root causes through natural mechanisms. Here are several ways herbal medicine can help men suffering from ED:

1. Improving Blood Circulation

Erectile dysfunction is often linked to poor blood flow. For an erection to occur, blood must flow into the penis and stay there during sexual arousal. Herbs that enhance blood circulation improve this process naturally, without the need for synthetic medications.

- **Vasodilation**: Many herbs promote the dilation of blood vessels, allowing more blood to flow into the penis. For example, **ginkgo biloba** improves blood circulation by increasing the production of nitric oxide, which relaxes blood vessels.

- **Reducing oxidative stress**: Some herbal remedies, such as **ginseng** and **tribulus terrestris**, are known for their antioxidant properties. These herbs help reduce oxidative stress, which can damage blood vessels and impair circulation, leading to ED.

2. Balancing Hormones

Low testosterone levels or other hormonal imbalances are common causes of ED. Herbal medicine can help stimulate the production of key hormones like testosterone, which is essential for maintaining libido, erectile function, and overall sexual health.

- **Testosterone boosters**: Herbs like **maca root** and **fenugreek** have been used to naturally raise testosterone levels. Maca root, in particular, has been shown to enhance libido and sexual stamina, which may help combat ED.
- **Adaptogens**: Adaptogenic herbs such as **ashwagandha** and **rhodiola** support the body's ability to manage stress, which in turn helps balance hormone production. Ashwagandha, in particular, is known for its ability to lower cortisol levels, a stress hormone that can interfere with testosterone production.

3. Reducing Anxiety and Stress

Psychological factors, such as stress, anxiety, and depression, can contribute to ED. Herbal medicine provides natural remedies that alleviate stress and anxiety, which can help improve sexual performance.

- **Anxiolytic herbs**: Herbs like **valerian root** and **passionflower** have calming effects on the nervous system, which can help reduce anxiety and stress levels. By addressing these psychological barriers, they allow men to relax, which is essential for sexual arousal and performance.
- **Mood enhancers**: **St. John's Wort** and **kava** are herbs that have been traditionally used to treat depression and boost mood. By improving mental well-being, these herbs indirectly support sexual health.

4. Enhancing Libido and Sexual Stamina

Low libido is another common problem that accompanies erectile dysfunction. Some herbs are known for their aphrodisiac properties, which help stimulate sexual desire and improve performance.

- **Aphrodisiac herbs**: **Horny goat weed** (Epimedium) is one of the most well-known herbal remedies for sexual dysfunction. It contains the compound icariin, which works similarly to Viagra by inhibiting the enzyme that restricts blood flow to the penis.
- **Energy boosters**: Herbs like **ginseng** and **maca root** help boost energy and endurance, which can improve overall sexual stamina. Ginseng has been shown in several studies to have a positive impact on sexual arousal and satisfaction, making it a popular choice for men with ED.

5. Addressing Deficiencies

Nutritional deficiencies can contribute to erectile dysfunction, and herbal medicine can help by providing essential nutrients that the body may be lacking. Certain herbs are rich in vitamins, minerals, and amino acids that are crucial for sexual health.

- **Zinc deficiency**: Zinc is essential for testosterone production, and a deficiency in this mineral can lead to low libido and erectile dysfunction. Herbs like **fenugreek** are high in zinc and can help restore normal testosterone levels.

- **Magnesium deficiency**: Magnesium is important for regulating blood pressure and improving circulation. **Leafy green herbs** like parsley and nettle are high in magnesium and can help improve blood flow to the penis.

HERBAL MEDICINES THAT PROMOTE SEXUAL HEALTH

There are several herbs traditionally used to enhance sexual health and combat erectile dysfunction. Below are some of the most effective and widely studied herbal remedies:

1. Ginkgo Biloba

Ginkgo biloba is one of the most popular herbs for improving circulation, which is essential for erectile function. It enhances blood flow by increasing nitric oxide levels, helping to relax blood vessels and allowing more blood to flow into the penis.

- **Benefits**: Improves circulation, boosts libido, enhances memory, and reduces anxiety.
- **Deficiency**: Ginkgo may cause side effects in people taking blood thinners as it can

interact with these medications, leading to increased bleeding risk.

2. Panax Ginseng (Korean Red Ginseng)

Ginseng has been used for centuries in Chinese medicine to improve overall vitality and treat sexual dysfunction. Studies have shown that it can enhance erectile function by increasing nitric oxide production, reducing oxidative stress, and improving circulation.

- **Benefits**: Enhances stamina, reduces stress, boosts nitric oxide, and improves libido.
- **Deficiency**: Long-term use can cause headaches, insomnia, or digestive issues in some individuals.

3. Horny Goat Weed (Epimedium)

Horny goat weed is a traditional Chinese remedy that contains icariin, a compound that helps improve erectile function by increasing blood flow to the penis. It works by blocking the enzyme phosphodiesterase type 5 (PDE5), which is the same mechanism that prescription ED drugs like Viagra use.

- **Benefits**: Increases libido, improves erectile function, and boosts stamina.
- **Deficiency**: Potential side effects include dizziness, dry mouth, and nosebleeds.

4. Maca Root

Maca root, a plant native to the Andes, has been traditionally used to boost libido and enhance fertility. Maca is rich in essential nutrients that support hormone balance and improve energy levels, making it an excellent choice for men experiencing ED.

- **Benefits**: Increases libido, boosts stamina, supports hormone balance, and enhances mood.
- **Deficiency**: Rare side effects include digestive discomfort and insomnia, especially when taken in high doses.

5. Tribulus Terrestris

Tribulus terrestris is an herb commonly used in Ayurvedic and Traditional Chinese Medicine to enhance sexual performance and treat infertility. It is believed to work by increasing the body's natural testosterone levels, although more research is needed to confirm its effects.

- **Benefits**: Boosts testosterone levels, improves libido, and enhances sexual stamina.

- **Deficiency**: Can cause stomach upset, cramping, or skin reactions in some individuals.

6. Ashwagandha

Ashwagandha, also known as Indian ginseng, is an adaptogen that helps the body manage stress. It is particularly beneficial for men whose ED is linked to stress or anxiety, as it promotes relaxation and supports overall hormonal balance.

- **Benefits**: Reduces stress and anxiety, supports hormone balance, improves stamina, and boosts sexual function.
- **Deficiency**: Can cause drowsiness, digestive upset, or, in rare cases, allergic reactions.

7. Saw Palmetto

Saw palmetto is an herb known for supporting prostate health, which is directly linked to male sexual health. It is often used to treat benign prostatic hyperplasia (BPH), a condition that can cause ED in older men.

- **Benefits**: Supports prostate health, enhances libido, and improves sexual stamina.
- **Deficiency**: Some individuals may experience mild side effects like stomach pain or headaches.

Deficiencies and Effects of Herbal Medicine

While herbal remedies can be effective in treating erectile dysfunction, they are not without potential risks or deficiencies. It is essential to understand that:

- **Herbal medicines can interact with prescription drugs**: Some herbs, like ginkgo biloba or horny goat weed, can interact with medications such as blood thinners or drugs for high blood pressure. These interactions can cause harmful side effects, so it is important for patients to consult with a healthcare professional before starting any herbal treatment.

- **Lack of standardization**: Unlike pharmaceuticals, herbal supplements are not always subject to rigorous testing or standardization. This means that the potency and quality of herbal remedies can vary from one product to another, potentially affecting their effectiveness.

- **Delayed results**: Herbal treatments often require more time to show effects compared to prescription medications. Patients need to be consistent with their use and patient when it comes to seeing improvements.

- **Potential side effects**: While herbal remedies are natural, they are not necessarily free from side effects. Some herbs can cause digestive issues, allergic reactions, or other mild side effects, especially when taken in high doses.

GINKGO BILOBA IN TREATING ERECTILE DYSFUNCTION (ED)

Ginkgo biloba is one of the oldest living tree species in the world and has been used for centuries in traditional Chinese medicine. It is widely known for its potential to improve cognitive function, reduce anxiety, and support overall cardiovascular health. However, one of its lesser-known but highly significant benefits is its use in treating erectile dysfunction (ED).

Erectile dysfunction is a common condition that affects men's ability to achieve or maintain an erection. It is often linked to issues with blood flow, stress, anxiety, or underlying health conditions such as heart disease or diabetes. Ginkgo biloba, through its ability to improve blood circulation and act as an antioxidant, has emerged as a natural alternative or supplement to conventional ED treatments.

How Ginkgo Biloba Affects and Helps ED Patients

1. Improving Blood Circulation

One of the primary reasons for erectile dysfunction is insufficient blood flow to the penis. Erections occur when blood fills the penile tissue, but when blood vessels are narrowed or circulation is compromised due to conditions such as high blood pressure or cardiovascular disease, achieving an erection becomes difficult.

Ginkgo biloba has a well-documented effect on improving blood circulation. It helps dilate blood vessels, improving the flow of oxygenated blood throughout the body, including to the genital area. By increasing blood flow, Ginkgo biloba can help men with ED achieve and maintain an erection.

- **Mechanism**: Ginkgo biloba contains flavonoids and terpenoids, compounds

51

that act as vasodilators. These compounds help relax the smooth muscles of the blood vessels, improving overall circulation and allowing for better blood flow to the penis during sexual arousal.

2. Enhancing Nitric Oxide Levels

Nitric oxide is a crucial molecule in the process of achieving an erection. It helps relax the blood vessels and improves blood flow to the penis, a key factor in maintaining an erection. Ginkgo biloba has been shown to enhance the release of nitric oxide, supporting vascular relaxation and thereby improving erectile function.

- **Research Evidence**: Several studies suggest that Ginkgo biloba can improve erectile function, especially in cases where ED is caused by vascular issues. A study published in the "Journal of Urology" showed that Ginkgo biloba improved blood flow and helped treat ED, especially in men who had ED related to antidepressant medications.

3. Reducing Anxiety and Stress

Psychological factors such as stress and anxiety are major contributors to erectile dysfunction. Performance anxiety, for instance, can lead to a cycle where worry over achieving an erection causes continued problems with sexual performance.

Ginkgo biloba has natural anti-anxiety properties that may help alleviate these psychological barriers to sexual function. By reducing stress and anxiety, it can create a more relaxed mental state, which is essential for sexual arousal and erectile function.

- **Mechanism**: Ginkgo biloba works by balancing cortisol levels and improving the body's response to stress. Additionally, it has been shown to have mild sedative effects, helping men relax mentally and emotionally, which can lead to better sexual performance.

4. Supporting Libido and Sexual Desire

Apart from its direct effect on circulation and mental relaxation, Ginkgo biloba has been associated with an increase in sexual desire or libido. This may be due to the herb's overall impact on energy levels, mood stabilization, and enhancement of overall vitality. For men suffering from low libido, especially those with ED caused by stress or anxiety, Ginkgo biloba can offer both psychological and physiological benefits.

Ginkgo Biloba's Role in Promoting Sexual Health

While Ginkgo biloba is primarily known for its circulatory and mental health benefits, its positive effects on sexual health are becoming increasingly recognized. Here are some of the ways Ginkgo biloba promotes overall sexual health:

1. Improves Cardiovascular Health

Since cardiovascular health is closely linked to sexual function, improving heart health naturally enhances sexual performance. Ginkgo biloba's ability to improve blood vessel health and reduce inflammation means that it supports both heart and sexual health in tandem. This is especially beneficial for men with ED linked to cardiovascular issues, as improved circulation can also benefit heart function.

2. Boosts Energy and Stamina

Chronic fatigue and low energy levels can impact libido and sexual performance. Ginkgo biloba, by improving oxygen delivery and blood flow, can increase energy levels and stamina. This effect contributes to more sustained sexual performance and higher sexual satisfaction.

3. Antioxidant Properties

Ginkgo biloba contains powerful antioxidants that neutralize free radicals in the body. Free radicals are unstable molecules that can cause oxidative stress, damaging tissues and accelerating aging. By reducing oxidative stress, Ginkgo biloba helps protect cells from damage, including those in the reproductive system, promoting long-term sexual health.

4. Enhances Cognitive Function

Sexual performance is often tied to mental focus and mood. Ginkgo biloba's ability to enhance cognitive function and improve memory can lead to more clarity of thought and better mental engagement in intimate situations.

Ginkgo Biloba Recipe for ED Support: Preparation at Home

Incorporating Ginkgo biloba into your daily routine to support erectile function can be done with simple homemade remedies. Below is a recipe for making Ginkgo biloba tea, a popular way to consume the herb and benefit from its health-boosting properties.

GINKGO BILOBA TEA RECIPE

Ingredients:

- 1 teaspoon of dried Ginkgo biloba leaves (you can find these in health food stores or online, or harvest and dry your own from a Ginkgo tree)

- 1 cup of water
- Honey or lemon (optional, for taste)

Directions:

1. Boil one cup of water in a kettle or pot.
2. Place 1 teaspoon of dried Ginkgo biloba leaves in a teapot or mug.
3. Pour the hot water over the Ginkgo biloba leaves.
4. Cover the pot or mug and allow the leaves to steep for 5-10 minutes.
5. Strain the tea to remove the leaves.
6. Optional: Add honey or lemon for flavor if desired.
7. Enjoy the tea warm.

Dosage: Drink one cup of Ginkgo biloba tea per day to promote circulation and sexual health. If you are using Ginkgo biloba supplements (such as capsules or tinctures), follow the dosage instructions on the product packaging, or consult a healthcare provider.

Considerations and Precautions

While Ginkgo biloba is generally considered safe for most people, there are a few considerations to keep in mind, especially if you are using it for erectile dysfunction:

1. **Consult a Doctor**: Before starting Ginkgo biloba, particularly if you are already on medication for ED, blood pressure, or heart conditions, consult with a healthcare professional. Ginkgo biloba can interact with blood-thinning medications or other treatments.

2. **Potential Side Effects**: Though rare, some people may experience mild side effects such as headaches, dizziness, or stomach upset when taking Ginkgo biloba. It is

important to start with a small dose to see how your body reacts.

3. **Consistency Is Key**: The effects of Ginkgo biloba on ED are not immediate. Like many herbal remedies, it may take several weeks or even months of consistent use to see noticeable improvements in erectile function and sexual health.

Ginkgo biloba has emerged as a natural and effective supplement for erectile dysfunction due to its ability to improve blood circulation, enhance nitric oxide levels, and reduce stress. By promoting healthy blood flow and alleviating psychological stressors, Ginkgo biloba supports both the physical and mental aspects of sexual performance. With its wide range of additional health benefits, such as boosting cognitive function and protecting against oxidative damage, this ancient herb offers a holistic approach to sexual health.

Incorporating Ginkgo biloba into your daily routine through tea or supplements may offer a natural solution to ED while promoting overall well-being. Whether as a standalone treatment or a supplement to traditional ED therapies, Ginkgo biloba can play a significant role in improving sexual health and performance.

PANAX GINSENG (KOREAN RED GINSENG) IN ERECTILE DYSFUNCTION

Panax ginseng, often referred to as Korean Red Ginseng, is a widely used herbal remedy for a variety of health conditions, including sexual health problems like erectile dysfunction (ED). It has been used for centuries in traditional Chinese and Korean medicine for its potent medicinal properties, particularly its ability to promote vitality, enhance stamina, and improve overall well-being. Scientific studies over the years have supported the use of Panax ginseng as a natural treatment for erectile dysfunction, making it a popular herbal supplement for improving male sexual health.

Understanding Erectile Dysfunction and How Panax Ginseng Can Help

Erectile dysfunction occurs when there is an inability to achieve or sustain an erection firm enough for sexual intercourse. ED is often caused by a combination of physical and psychological factors, such as cardiovascular issues, poor blood circulation, hormone imbalances, stress, anxiety, and aging.

Panax ginseng is considered an **adaptogen**, meaning it helps the body resist stress and improve overall health, making it a holistic option for treating erectile dysfunction. It is known for its ability to **enhance nitric oxide production, improve circulation, and promote energy levels**, all of which play a crucial role in sexual health. The root contains **ginsenosides**, which are active compounds believed to be responsible for its various health benefits, including its effects on erectile function.

Benefits of Panax Ginseng for Erectile Dysfunction

Several studies have shown that Panax ginseng can significantly improve erectile function, especially in men with mild to moderate ED. Here are some of the key ways it helps erectile dysfunction patients:

1. Improving Nitric Oxide Production

Nitric oxide is a crucial molecule that helps relax the smooth muscles in the penis, allowing blood to flow into the erectile tissues. Adequate blood flow is essential for achieving and maintaining an erection. One of the most significant ways Panax ginseng helps with ED is by **enhancing nitric oxide production**, which improves blood circulation and ensures that the erectile tissues receive sufficient blood flow.

In a study published in the *Journal of Urology*, men with ED who took Panax ginseng saw significant improvement in erectile function, likely due to the ginsenosides stimulating the production of nitric oxide, which enhances vascular function.

2. Boosting Energy and Stamina

One of the hallmarks of Panax ginseng is its ability to boost energy and reduce fatigue. Ginseng helps improve physical stamina, reduce feelings of fatigue, and enhance mental alertness. This is particularly beneficial for individuals experiencing ED related to exhaustion or low energy levels. By improving overall vitality, ginseng helps men sustain the physical energy required for sexual activity.

3. Hormonal Balance

Panax ginseng has been shown to have a **positive effect on testosterone levels**, which are critical for male sexual health. Testosterone influences libido, sperm production, and overall erectile function. Studies suggest that ginsenosides in ginseng help modulate hormonal balance, which may improve sexual desire and performance in men suffering from low testosterone or hormonal imbalances.

4. Reducing Stress and Anxiety

Psychological factors like stress, anxiety, and depression are common causes of ED. Panax ginseng is known for its **adaptogenic properties**, meaning it helps the body adapt to stress by balancing the release of cortisol and other stress hormones. This reduction in stress and anxiety can have a direct impact on sexual performance, as men are more likely to experience ED when they are tense or mentally fatigued.

A reduction in stress hormones also allows the body to prioritize blood flow and energy toward physical performance, including sexual activity.

5. Improving Circulation and Cardiovascular Health

Since ED is often related to cardiovascular problems, improving heart health and circulation can help alleviate symptoms of ED. Panax ginseng is known to promote cardiovascular health by **reducing inflammation, lowering cholesterol levels, and improving blood vessel function**. By supporting better circulation, ginseng can indirectly improve erectile function and help with conditions like atherosclerosis, which often contributes to ED.

How Panax Ginseng Promotes Sexual Health

Beyond just treating erectile dysfunction, Panax ginseng supports overall sexual health in various ways:

1. **Increased Libido**: Many men experience an increase in sexual desire after regularly consuming Panax ginseng. This is likely due to its effects on energy levels, hormonal balance, and overall vitality.

2. **Better Sperm Quality**: Studies have shown that Panax ginseng may help improve sperm motility and quality, making it beneficial for men struggling with infertility or suboptimal sperm parameters.

3. **Improved Sexual Confidence**: By enhancing energy, reducing stress, and improving blood flow, Panax ginseng can contribute to a man's confidence in his

sexual performance, which plays a key role in sexual health and satisfaction.

RECIPE AND PREPARATION OF PANAX GINSENG (KOREAN RED GINSENG) AT HOME

Panax ginseng can be consumed in various forms, including teas, tinctures, capsules, and powders. For those who prefer a natural, homemade preparation, **ginseng tea** is a popular and easy way to incorporate this powerful herb into a daily routine.

Ingredients:

- **3-5 grams of dried Korean Red Ginseng root** (you can find this at herbal shops or online)
- **2 cups of water**
- Optional: honey, lemon, or ginger for flavor

Preparation Instructions:

1. **Prepare the Ginseng Root**: If you have dried ginseng root, slice it thinly or use it whole. Some people prefer to grind the ginseng into a powder, but slices work well for tea.

2. **Boil Water**: Bring 2 cups of water to a boil in a small saucepan.

3. **Simmer the Ginseng**: Once the water is boiling, reduce the heat to a simmer and add the ginseng slices or powder. Let the ginseng simmer in the water for about **15-20 minutes**. The longer you simmer, the stronger the tea will become.

4. **Strain and Serve**: After simmering, strain the tea into a cup to remove the ginseng pieces. You can add honey, lemon, or ginger for added flavor, though the tea has a naturally earthy and slightly bitter taste.

5. **Drink Regularly**: For maximum benefits, drink ginseng tea **once or twice a day**.

Consistency is key, as the benefits of ginseng tend to build over time with regular use.

Optional: Ginseng Infused Honey Recipe

For those who prefer a sweeter preparation, you can make **ginseng-infused honey** that can be added to teas or consumed directly.

1. **Slice 3-5 grams of dried ginseng root** into thin pieces.
2. **Place the slices into a small jar** and cover with **raw honey**.
3. Let the honey infuse with ginseng for **at least 1-2 weeks**.
4. After infusing, the honey will take on the medicinal properties of ginseng and can be used in tea, on toast, or consumed by the spoonful for an energy boost and ED support.

Safety and Considerations

While Panax ginseng is generally considered safe, it is important to use it in moderation and consult with a healthcare provider before starting any herbal supplement, particularly for individuals with underlying health conditions or those taking medications. Ginseng may interact with blood pressure medications, insulin, and other pharmaceuticals, so it's essential to ensure it doesn't cause adverse effects.

Panax ginseng, particularly Korean Red Ginseng, has been shown to be an effective natural treatment for erectile dysfunction. Its ability to enhance nitric oxide production, improve circulation, balance hormones, and reduce stress makes it a comprehensive remedy for men suffering from ED. When combined with a healthy lifestyle and proper medical guidance, Panax ginseng can play a pivotal role in restoring sexual health, boosting energy, and improving overall vitality. Incorporating ginseng into the daily routine, whether through tea or other forms, offers a natural, time-tested method to support male sexual health.

HORNY GOAT WEED (EPIMEDIUM) FOR ERECTILE DYSFUNCTION

Horny Goat Weed, scientifically known as **Epimedium**, is a traditional herbal remedy that has been used for centuries in Chinese medicine to enhance sexual health, particularly for treating **erectile dysfunction (ED)**. The herb derives its interesting name from a legendary story in which a goat herder noticed increased sexual activity in his goats after they grazed on the Epimedium plant, leading to its reputation as a potent aphrodisiac.

Epimedium contains a powerful bioactive compound called **icariin**, which is thought to be the main active ingredient responsible for its beneficial effects on sexual health. Today, it is gaining popularity in modern natural medicine as a treatment for ED, often serving as a natural alternative to pharmaceuticals like Viagra.

The Role of Horny Goat Weed in Treating Erectile Dysfunction

Erectile dysfunction occurs when there is insufficient blood flow to the penis, preventing an erection firm enough for sexual activity. Several factors, including poor cardiovascular health, hormonal imbalances, stress, and even neurological conditions, can contribute to ED. Horny Goat Weed is believed to address these underlying causes by working in several ways to improve sexual function.

1. Boosting Nitric Oxide Levels

One of the primary mechanisms by which Horny Goat Weed improves erectile function is through its ability to enhance **nitric oxide** production. Nitric oxide is essential for vasodilation, a process where blood vessels relax and widen, allowing for increased blood flow. In the case of erectile dysfunction, nitric oxide allows blood to flow more easily to the penis, facilitating stronger and longer-lasting erections.

Icariin, the active compound in Horny Goat Weed, is believed to inhibit **phosphodiesterase type 5 (PDE5)**, an enzyme that restricts blood flow to the penis. This inhibition mirrors the action of pharmaceutical drugs like Viagra and Cialis, which are PDE5 inhibitors. By inhibiting PDE5, icariin increases nitric oxide levels, thereby improving blood flow and erectile function.

2. Balancing Hormones and Boosting Libido

Horny Goat Weed has been shown to influence hormone levels, particularly **testosterone**, which plays a key role in male sexual health. Testosterone is critical for libido (sex drive), energy levels, and the ability to achieve an erection. As men age, testosterone levels naturally decline, leading to diminished sexual desire and performance.

Several studies suggest that Horny Goat Weed can help increase testosterone production, enhancing libido and overall sexual performance. This boost in testosterone may also contribute to improved mood, energy, and stamina—all factors that can positively impact sexual health.

3. Reducing Stress and Fatigue

Stress, anxiety, and fatigue are major contributors to erectile dysfunction. The icariin found in Horny Goat Weed has adaptogenic properties, which means it helps the body manage and adapt to stress. By promoting a sense of calm and reducing anxiety, Horny Goat Weed helps alleviate the mental barriers that often accompany erectile dysfunction.

Additionally, the herb's ability to combat fatigue can enhance physical endurance, contributing to better sexual performance and energy levels.

4. Enhancing Overall Circulation

Good circulation is essential not just for erectile function but for overall health. Horny Goat Weed improves circulation by promoting better blood flow throughout the body. Its vasodilatory effects can help prevent cardiovascular issues that may contribute to ED, making it a heart-healthy herb as well.

5. Neurological Health

Some research suggests that icariin may have neuroprotective effects, meaning it can protect nerve cells from damage. This is important because ED can sometimes be caused by neurological issues, such as damage to the nerves responsible for sending signals between the brain and the penis. By improving nerve health, Horny Goat Weed may help improve the communication between the brain and the genitals, resulting in better erectile function.

The Importance of Horny Goat Weed for Erectile Dysfunction Patients

For men dealing with erectile dysfunction, Horny Goat Weed offers a natural alternative to pharmaceutical treatments. It may be particularly appealing for those looking to avoid the side effects of conventional ED medications, which can include headaches, dizziness, and digestive issues.

Unlike synthetic drugs that only treat the symptoms of ED, Horny Goat Weed works holistically, addressing the root causes of erectile dysfunction, such as poor circulation, hormonal imbalances, and stress. This makes it a versatile solution for promoting sexual health and improving overall well-being.

Horny Goat Weed also comes with a range of additional health benefits. Aside from its role in sexual health, it has been used to improve bone density, enhance immune function, and alleviate symptoms of menopause. This makes it a powerful adaptogen with wide-ranging health benefits beyond just treating ED.

How Horny Goat Weed Promotes Sexual Health

1. **Increased Blood Flow:** By boosting nitric oxide production, Horny Goat Weed improves circulation to the penis, resulting in stronger erections.

2. **Hormonal Support:** The herb can help increase testosterone levels, which supports sexual desire and performance.

3. **Stress Reduction:** Its adaptogenic properties help combat stress, anxiety, and fatigue, all of which can impair sexual function.

4. **Enhanced Libido:** Horny Goat Weed has a long history of use as an aphrodisiac, enhancing sexual desire and pleasure.

5. **Support for Nerve Health:** Icariin's neuroprotective qualities may help improve communication between the brain and penis, supporting better erectile function.

A Recipe and Preparation of Horny Goat Weed (Epimedium) at Home

Horny Goat Weed is widely available as a supplement, but it can also be prepared at home in the form of tea, tincture, or extract. Below is a simple recipe to create your own Horny Goat Weed infusion at home.

HORNY GOAT WEED TEA RECIPE
Ingredients:

- 1 to 2 teaspoons of dried **Horny Goat Weed (Epimedium)** leaves (available at herbal stores or online)
- 2 cups of filtered water
- Optional: honey or lemon for flavor

Directions:

1. **Boil the water**: Bring 2 cups of water to a rolling boil in a pot or kettle.
2. **Steep the leaves**: Place the dried Horny Goat Weed leaves in a teapot or heat-resistant container. Pour the boiling water over the leaves.
3. **Steep for 5-10 minutes**: Allow the leaves to steep for at least 5 minutes. For a

stronger brew, steep for 10 minutes, but avoid going beyond this, as it may result in a bitter taste.

4. **Strain the tea**: Using a fine mesh strainer, pour the tea into a mug, straining out the leaves.

5. **Add flavor**: If desired, add a teaspoon of honey or a slice of lemon for flavor. These will also provide additional health benefits such as antioxidant and anti-inflammatory properties.

6. **Drink warm**: Sip the tea slowly while warm. Horny Goat Weed tea can be consumed 1-2 times daily to improve sexual health.

Homemade Horny Goat Weed Tincture

Tinctures are a potent way to extract the active compounds from Horny Goat Weed, and they offer a more concentrated form of the herb than tea.

Ingredients:

- 1 cup of dried **Horny Goat Weed** leaves
- 2 cups of high-proof vodka or brandy (at least 80 proof)
- A glass jar with a tight-fitting lid
- Cheesecloth or fine strainer
- Dropper bottle

Directions:

1. **Prepare the leaves**: Place 1 cup of dried Horny Goat Weed leaves into a clean glass jar.
2. **Add the alcohol**: Pour 2 cups of vodka or brandy over the leaves, ensuring that the leaves are fully submerged.
3. **Seal the jar**: Place the lid on the jar tightly and shake well.

4. **Store and steep**: Store the jar in a cool, dark place for 4-6 weeks, shaking it daily to help with the extraction process.

5. **Strain the mixture**: After 4-6 weeks, strain the tincture using cheesecloth or a fine mesh strainer. Transfer the liquid to a clean glass bottle or dropper bottle for storage.

6. **Dosage**: Start by taking 1-2 droppers full (about 20-40 drops) under the tongue, once or twice daily. Tinctures can also be added to water or juice.

Horny Goat Weed (Epimedium) offers a powerful, natural solution for erectile dysfunction and other sexual health issues. Its ability to increase blood flow, boost testosterone, reduce stress, and enhance libido makes it an excellent remedy for those seeking an alternative to synthetic medications.

MACA ROOT AND ERECTILE DYSFUNCTION

Maca root (Lepidium meyenii) is a plant native to the Andes mountains of Peru, revered for its ability to improve stamina, energy, and fertility. Historically used by the Inca civilization for both culinary and medicinal purposes, maca has been gaining popularity worldwide for its potential benefits in sexual health, especially in addressing issues like erectile dysfunction (ED). Maca root is often referred to as "Peruvian ginseng," though it belongs to the cruciferous family, which includes broccoli and cauliflower.

The Role of Maca Root in Addressing Erectile Dysfunction

Erectile dysfunction, the inability to achieve or maintain an erection, can be caused by a variety of factors, such as poor blood circulation, hormone imbalances, psychological stress, and lifestyle choices. Maca root has been widely studied for its aphrodisiac properties, and its potential role in improving sexual performance, stamina, and libido makes it an appealing natural remedy for men struggling with ED.

Maca root does not directly affect the body's hormonal system like synthetic ED medications (e.g., Viagra), but it works in a holistic manner, supporting overall health and vitality, which can lead to improved sexual function.

How Maca Root Affects Erectile Dysfunction Patients

1. **Enhances Libido and Sexual Desire:** One of the most well-documented benefits of maca root is its ability to enhance libido. Various studies have shown that regular consumption of maca can significantly

increase sexual desire in men, which is a key factor for those suffering from erectile dysfunction. Maca's aphrodisiac properties are thought to be linked to its ability to boost energy levels, reduce anxiety, and increase overall well-being, which may directly influence sexual desire.

In a study published in *Andrologia* in 2009, men who took maca supplements experienced a notable increase in sexual desire compared to those who took a placebo, indicating maca's potential to enhance libido without affecting testosterone levels.

2. **Improves Blood Circulation:** Poor blood circulation is a leading cause of erectile dysfunction, as the inability to supply sufficient blood to the penis prevents a firm erection. Maca root contains

compounds that can improve cardiovascular health, which in turn boosts blood flow throughout the body, including to the pelvic area. By improving circulation, maca can help men achieve stronger and more sustainable erections.

3. **Supports Hormonal Balance:** While maca does not directly influence testosterone levels, it does play a role in balancing hormones. Maca acts as an adaptogen, meaning it helps the body adapt to stress and supports the endocrine system. This balance of hormones is crucial for sexual health, as imbalances in cortisol (the stress hormone), estrogen, and testosterone can contribute to erectile dysfunction. In particular, cortisol is known to interfere with sexual performance, and maca's ability to reduce stress may have a positive impact on ED.

4. **Increases Energy and Reduces Fatigue:** Many men suffering from ED also struggle with fatigue, low energy, or low stamina. Maca root is often used as a natural energy booster and has been shown to improve endurance and reduce feelings of fatigue. The root is rich in essential nutrients, including vitamins B, C, and E, which contribute to increased vitality. Enhanced energy levels can lead to improved physical performance, including in sexual activities.

5. **Reduces Psychological Stress and Anxiety:** Erectile dysfunction is often linked to psychological factors such as stress, depression, and anxiety. Maca root has adaptogenic properties, helping the body cope with stress and promoting mental clarity. Studies have shown that maca can reduce symptoms of anxiety and

depression, which in turn can alleviate the psychological barriers that contribute to ED.

6. **Promotes General Sexual Health:** Maca root contains a variety of nutrients that contribute to sexual health, including protein, fiber, and essential amino acids. These nutrients not only improve stamina and energy but also enhance reproductive function. Additionally, maca has been shown to increase sperm production and improve sperm motility, further supporting male reproductive health.

How Maca Root Promotes Sexual Health

Maca is rich in phytonutrients, antioxidants, and unique compounds that are beneficial for overall health and specifically sexual health. Some key elements of maca's contribution to sexual well-being include:

1. **Alkaloids:** These compounds in maca help stimulate the hypothalamus and pituitary gland, both of which are critical for hormone regulation.

2. **Glucosinolates:** Maca contains glucosinolates, which have been linked to cancer prevention but also contribute to hormonal balance, potentially enhancing sexual function.

3. **Lepidium Sterols:** Sterols found in maca can support male reproductive health by potentially increasing libido, sperm health, and sexual stamina.

4. **Nutrients:** Maca is rich in vitamins (such as B6, C, and E), minerals (calcium, magnesium, potassium), and essential fatty acids, all of which are essential for overall health and sexual wellness.

PREPARING "HORNY MACA ROOT" AT HOME

You can easily prepare a maca-infused drink at home to boost your sexual health naturally. Here's a simple recipe that incorporates maca powder, designed to enhance energy, improve libido, and support erectile function.

Ingredients:

- 1 teaspoon maca root powder (available at health food stores)
- 1 tablespoon raw cacao powder (optional, adds flavor and enhances circulation)
- 1 cup almond milk (or any plant-based milk)
- 1 tablespoon honey or maple syrup (for sweetness)
- 1/2 teaspoon cinnamon (promotes circulation and adds a warming effect)
- 1/4 teaspoon ground ginger (enhances blood flow)

- 1/4 teaspoon vanilla extract (optional, for flavor)
- Ice cubes (optional for a cold version)

Directions:

1. **Heat the Almond Milk**: In a small saucepan, warm the almond milk over medium heat until it is just about to simmer. You can also serve this drink cold by skipping this step and blending the ingredients with ice instead.
2. **Mix the Powders**: In a small bowl, combine the maca root powder, raw cacao powder (if using), cinnamon, and ginger.
3. **Blend the Ingredients**: Slowly whisk the powder mixture into the warmed almond milk, ensuring there are no clumps. Continue to stir until fully blended and smooth.

4. **Sweeten the Drink**: Add the honey or maple syrup to taste and whisk until the sweetener is dissolved.

5. **Add Vanilla (Optional)**: Stir in the vanilla extract for an extra layer of flavor.

6. **Serve**: Pour the maca root drink into a mug if serving warm, or over ice in a glass if you prefer it cold. Enjoy!

Optional Boosters:

- **Chia Seeds**: For added nutrition, you can blend in a teaspoon of chia seeds, which are high in omega-3 fatty acids and promote heart health.

- **MCT Oil**: Add a teaspoon of MCT oil for a quick energy boost.

Benefits of Horny Maca Root Drink:

- This maca drink boosts energy levels, helps combat fatigue, and improves stamina, making it ideal for enhancing sexual performance.

- The combination of maca, cacao, and warming spices like cinnamon and ginger promotes better circulation, which is essential for addressing ED.
- The drink is a natural aphrodisiac that supports overall sexual health by balancing hormones and improving mental clarity.

Maca root offers a natural, holistic approach to managing erectile dysfunction by addressing both the physical and psychological factors that contribute to the condition. By enhancing energy levels, improving blood circulation, balancing hormones, and reducing stress, maca provides a sustainable solution that can promote long-term sexual health and vitality

TRIBULUS TERRESTRIS FOR ERECTILE DYSFUNCTION (ED)

Tribulus Terrestris, a small leafy plant found in various parts of the world, is often associated with traditional medicine, especially in Ayurveda and Traditional Chinese Medicine. It has gained popularity in modern times for its reputed benefits in enhancing male sexual health, particularly for improving erectile dysfunction (ED). The active compounds in Tribulus Terrestris, particularly the saponins such as protodioscin, are believed to be responsible for its positive effects on libido, erectile function, and overall sexual well-being.

Understanding Erectile Dysfunction (ED) and Its Link to Tribulus Terrestris

Erectile dysfunction occurs when a man is unable to achieve or maintain an erection sufficient for sexual performance. The causes can be both physical and psychological, including poor blood flow, hormonal imbalances, stress, anxiety, and conditions like diabetes or cardiovascular diseases.

Tribulus Terrestris has been studied for its potential to address some of these underlying causes, especially concerning testosterone levels, blood circulation, and sexual desire. Here's how this plant works in relation to ED:

1. Increases Testosterone Levels

Testosterone, the primary male sex hormone, plays a crucial role in sexual health, libido, and erectile function. Low testosterone levels can lead to reduced sexual desire and erectile dysfunction. Tribulus Terrestris is believed to increase testosterone production by stimulating the pituitary gland to release luteinizing hormone

(LH), which signals the testes to produce more testosterone.

While some studies have shown that Tribulus Terrestris can increase testosterone levels in animals, research on humans is more varied. However, it is widely accepted that the plant helps with libido enhancement, even if its direct effect on testosterone in humans is still debated.

2. Enhances Libido and Sexual Desire

One of the most well-known benefits of Tribulus Terrestris is its ability to improve sexual desire or libido. For men with ED, a decreased libido can further complicate the condition, leading to psychological stress and performance anxiety. Tribulus Terrestris contains protodioscin, a steroidal saponin that enhances nitric oxide release, which improves blood flow to the genital area. Increased nitric oxide production also promotes a more relaxed state of the blood vessels, crucial for maintaining an erection.

Many studies have demonstrated that Tribulus Terrestris enhances sexual desire and satisfaction, making it useful for men with ED who struggle with low libido.

3. Improves Circulation and Blood Flow

Poor blood flow is a major contributor to ED, especially in men with cardiovascular conditions or diabetes. Tribulus Terrestris promotes better circulation by increasing the production of nitric oxide in the body. Nitric oxide acts as a vasodilator, relaxing the blood vessels and improving blood flow to the penile area. This mechanism is vital for achieving and maintaining an erection.

Improved circulation also benefits the entire body, promoting overall vitality and energy, which indirectly supports sexual performance.

4. Reduces Stress and Anxiety

Psychological factors such as stress, depression, and anxiety are common triggers of ED. Tribulus Terrestris has adaptogenic properties, which means it helps the body cope with stress by normalizing physiological functions. By reducing stress, Tribulus Terrestris indirectly improves sexual function and performance. The reduction of anxiety and the balancing of cortisol levels (the stress hormone) may help men experience fewer psychological barriers to sexual activity.

5. Supports Overall Reproductive Health

In addition to its benefits for erectile dysfunction, Tribulus Terrestris is also known to improve overall reproductive health. It has been used to treat conditions like infertility and low sperm count in men. Some research suggests that Tribulus Terrestris can enhance sperm motility and increase sperm count, making it a valuable natural remedy for men facing reproductive challenges.

How Tribulus Terrestris Promotes Sexual Health

Tribulus Terrestris contains various bioactive compounds, including flavonoids, alkaloids, and saponins. These compounds work synergistically to support sexual health in the following ways:

1. **Boosts Sexual Stamina and Performance**: Tribulus Terrestris may enhance stamina by improving energy levels and reducing fatigue, allowing men to engage in prolonged sexual activity.

2. **Balances Hormonal Levels**: By supporting testosterone production and regulating

other hormonal imbalances, Tribulus Terrestris promotes optimal sexual health. This balance is essential for both libido and erectile function.

3. **Natural Aphrodisiac**: In various traditional medicine systems, Tribulus Terrestris has been used as a natural aphrodisiac to increase sexual desire and treat impotence. Its ability to stimulate sexual arousal makes it particularly useful for men suffering from reduced libido due to stress, hormonal imbalances, or age.

4. **Increases Sensitivity and Sexual Satisfaction**: Improved blood flow to the genitals not only helps with erections but also enhances sensitivity and sexual pleasure. Men using Tribulus Terrestris may experience greater sexual satisfaction, both physically and emotionally.

TRIBULUS TERRESTRIS ROOT RECIPE AND PREPARATION AT HOME

Tribulus Terrestris can be consumed in various forms, such as powders, capsules, and tinctures. However, using the root of Tribulus Terrestris to make a tea or infusion is a traditional and effective way to reap its benefits.

Ingredients:

- 1 tablespoon dried Tribulus Terrestris root (available in herbal stores or online)
- 2 cups of water
- Honey or lemon (optional, for taste)

Instructions:

1. **Prepare the Root**: If using dried Tribulus Terrestris root, ensure it is clean and chopped into small pieces. You can also grind it slightly to release more of its active compounds.

2. **Boil the Water**: In a small pot, bring 2 cups of water to a boil.

3. **Simmer the Root**: Once the water is boiling, add 1 tablespoon of the dried Tribulus Terrestris root to the pot. Reduce the heat to a simmer.

4. **Steep**: Let the root steep in the simmering water for about 15-20 minutes. The longer it steeps, the stronger the tea will be. Make sure not to let it boil for too long, as this could break down the beneficial compounds.

5. **Strain**: After steeping, strain the tea into a cup to remove the root pieces.

6. **Add Honey or Lemon (Optional)**: If the tea tastes too bitter, you can add a bit of honey or lemon to enhance the flavor.

7. **Drink**: For best results, drink this tea once or twice a day. You can store the extra tea

in the refrigerator for up to 24 hours, but it is best consumed fresh.

Benefits of Tribulus Terrestris Tea:

- Boosts libido and enhances sexual performance.
- Improves energy levels and reduces fatigue.
- Supports hormonal balance and testosterone production.
- Promotes better blood circulation, which helps with erectile function.

Precautions and Considerations

While Tribulus Terrestris is generally considered safe, it is essential to consult a healthcare professional before starting any herbal remedy, especially if you have underlying health conditions or are taking other medications. Some individuals may experience mild side effects such as stomach upset, and in rare cases, it could interfere with medications, particularly those used to treat heart conditions or hormonal therapies.

Additionally, excessive use of Tribulus Terrestris over an extended period is not recommended, as it could cause hormonal imbalances. Moderation and monitoring are key to safe usage.

Tribulus Terrestris has a rich history of being used as a natural remedy for erectile dysfunction and male sexual health. Its ability to boost testosterone levels, enhance blood flow, reduce stress, and improve libido makes it a valuable herbal option for men seeking a natural alternative to pharmaceutical treatments. Whether consumed as a supplement or prepared at home in tea form, Tribulus Terrestris can provide a holistic and effective approach to improving erectile dysfunction and promoting overall sexual health.

ASHWAGANDHA

Ashwagandha, scientifically known as *Withania somnifera*, is a powerful adaptogenic herb that has been used for centuries in traditional Ayurvedic medicine. Known for its stress-relieving properties and ability to enhance overall vitality, Ashwagandha is gaining widespread recognition for its potential benefits in treating erectile dysfunction (ED) and promoting sexual health. Erectile dysfunction often stems from a combination of physical, hormonal, and psychological factors, and Ashwagandha's holistic approach to balancing these aspects makes it a natural choice for those seeking to address ED without relying on pharmaceuticals.

Role of Ashwagandha for Erectile Dysfunction

Erectile dysfunction can be caused by a variety of issues, including poor circulation, low testosterone levels, stress, and anxiety. Ashwagandha helps address these factors through its adaptogenic properties, meaning it helps the body adapt to stress and restore balance. Let's dive into the key ways in which Ashwagandha impacts erectile dysfunction:

1. Reduces Stress and Anxiety

One of the leading causes of ED, especially in younger men, is psychological stress. Anxiety, performance pressure, and chronic stress elevate cortisol levels, a hormone that disrupts the body's natural balance. Elevated cortisol can lower testosterone levels, impede blood flow, and increase the risk of ED.

Ashwagandha has been shown to reduce cortisol levels significantly. It works by calming the nervous system and promoting a sense of relaxation, which can alleviate the mental and emotional strain that often leads to ED. By helping men manage stress, Ashwagandha allows for better sexual performance and reduces psychological barriers to achieving and maintaining an erection.

A study published in the *Indian Journal of Psychological Medicine* found that Ashwagandha reduced cortisol levels by up to 28% in individuals who took the supplement regularly, showcasing its stress-lowering effects.

2. Improves Circulation and Blood Flow

Poor circulation is a major contributor to erectile dysfunction. For an erection to occur, there must be adequate blood flow to the penis. Ashwagandha supports cardiovascular health and improves blood circulation, particularly in the pelvic region, which is crucial for combating ED.

Ashwagandha is rich in antioxidants, which help to relax the blood vessels and reduce oxidative stress, improving overall blood flow. Its role in increasing nitric oxide production, a compound that dilates blood vessels, can significantly enhance erectile function by promoting better circulation.

3. Boosts Testosterone Levels

Low testosterone levels, or *hypogonadism*, are often linked to sexual dysfunction, including a decrease in libido and difficulty achieving erections. Ashwagandha has been shown to naturally boost testosterone levels, thereby improving sexual health.

In a clinical study, men who took Ashwagandha supplements experienced a significant increase in testosterone production compared to those who did not. Another study published in the *Journal of the International Society of Sports Nutrition* found that men who took Ashwagandha saw a 17% increase in testosterone levels and enhanced muscle strength and recovery, all of which positively impact sexual performance.

Higher testosterone levels improve not only libido but also energy levels, confidence, and sexual stamina, all of which can help men suffering from ED.

4. Enhances Overall Sexual Health and Vitality

Ashwagandha is considered a natural aphrodisiac in Ayurvedic medicine. By improving energy, reducing fatigue, and balancing hormones, it boosts libido and overall sexual satisfaction. Additionally, it promotes mental clarity and helps reduce mental fatigue, which can sometimes impede sexual desire.

For men who experience sexual dysfunction related to aging or fatigue, Ashwagandha provides a natural boost, enhancing sexual vitality and endurance. Studies also show that Ashwagandha can improve sperm quality and motility, making it beneficial for those dealing with fertility issues.

Importance of Ashwagandha for ED Patients

Ashwagandha's importance for men suffering from erectile dysfunction lies in its comprehensive approach to healing the body. Unlike synthetic drugs such as Viagra, which only provide temporary relief by increasing blood flow, Ashwagandha addresses the root causes of ED, including stress, hormonal imbalances, and poor circulation.

It is a natural, long-term solution that improves sexual health without the side effects associated with prescription medications. Since

Ashwagandha works gradually to restore balance in the body, it promotes sustainable sexual health rather than a short-term fix.

How Ashwagandha Promotes Sexual Health

- **Boosts Libido**: Regular consumption of Ashwagandha helps increase libido and sexual desire, thanks to its hormone-balancing properties and stress-reducing effects.

- **Increases Stamina**: Ashwagandha enhances endurance and stamina, both of which are crucial for improved sexual performance.

- **Reduces Erectile Dysfunction Symptoms**: By lowering stress and increasing nitric oxide levels, Ashwagandha can naturally alleviate some of the common symptoms of ED, such as difficulty maintaining an erection.

- **Improves Mood and Well-Being**: Sexual health is deeply connected to emotional and mental well-being. Ashwagandha improves mood by reducing anxiety, depression, and mental fatigue, all of which can contribute to a more fulfilling sex life.

- **Supports Hormonal Balance**: By promoting testosterone production and improving sperm quality, Ashwagandha ensures that the body's hormones are in balance, further supporting sexual health.

RECIPE AND PREPARATION OF ASHWAGANDHA ROOT AT HOME

Ashwagandha root can be prepared in a variety of ways to promote sexual health and overall well-being. Here's a simple recipe to create a homemade Ashwagandha root tonic that can be consumed regularly.

Ingredients:

- **Ashwagandha root powder**: 1 teaspoon
- **Water or milk (preferably almond or coconut milk)**: 1 cup
- **Honey** (optional, for sweetness): 1 teaspoon
- **Cinnamon or cardamom powder** (optional, for flavor): ¼ teaspoon
- **Ghee or coconut oil** (optional, for enhanced absorption of nutrients): ½ teaspoon

Preparation:

1. **Prepare the Ashwagandha Powder**: If you have whole Ashwagandha roots, you'll need to dry them thoroughly and grind them into a fine powder. Alternatively, you can buy Ashwagandha root powder from a reputable source.

2. **Boil the Liquid**: Heat the water or milk in a small saucepan until it begins to boil. If using water, you may want to add a bit of fat (like ghee or coconut oil), as it helps in the absorption of Ashwagandha's beneficial compounds.

3. **Add the Ashwagandha Powder**: Once the liquid is boiling, reduce the heat and stir in 1 teaspoon of Ashwagandha root powder. Let it simmer on low heat for about 5–10 minutes to extract the full medicinal properties of the herb.

4. **Add Sweeteners and Spices (Optional)**: If you prefer a slightly sweet flavor, stir in 1 teaspoon of honey or maple syrup after removing the mixture from heat. You can also add a dash of cinnamon or cardamom powder for additional flavor and health benefits.

5. **Serve Warm**: Pour the tonic into a cup and enjoy it warm, preferably in the evening before bedtime, as Ashwagandha can help relax the body and mind.

Dosage:

It is recommended to consume Ashwagandha tonic once or twice a day, depending on your body's needs and tolerance. You should start with a small amount (½ teaspoon) and gradually increase to 1 teaspoon daily to see how your body responds.

Ashwagandha offers a natural and effective solution for men dealing with erectile dysfunction by addressing the core issues of stress, poor circulation, and low testosterone levels. Its adaptogenic properties make it an excellent choice for promoting overall sexual health and vitality, while its holistic benefits extend to improving mood, reducing anxiety, and boosting stamina.

Incorporating Ashwagandha into your daily routine, through simple recipes like the Ashwagandha tonic, can be a valuable tool for improving sexual health naturally. By balancing hormones, enhancing blood flow, and reducing stress, Ashwagandha helps men achieve better sexual performance and long-term well-being.

SAW PALMETTO

Saw palmetto, derived from the fruit of the Serenoa repens plant, has gained popularity as a natural remedy for various health conditions, particularly those related to the prostate and sexual health. Traditionally used by Native American tribes and later in herbal medicine, saw palmetto is known for its potential benefits in promoting male reproductive health and addressing erectile dysfunction (ED).

The Role of Saw Palmetto in Erectile Dysfunction

1. **Hormonal Balance**:
   - Saw palmetto is thought to influence hormone levels in the body, particularly by inhibiting the conversion of testosterone to dihydrotestosterone (DHT). DHT is a potent androgen hormone that is

often linked to hair loss and can contribute to prostate enlargement. By reducing DHT levels, saw palmetto may help restore a healthy hormonal balance, which is crucial for sexual function.

o Hormonal imbalances, especially low testosterone levels, can lead to decreased libido and erectile dysfunction. By supporting testosterone levels, saw palmetto may indirectly enhance sexual desire and performance.

2. **Prostate Health**:

o An enlarged prostate (benign prostatic hyperplasia or BPH) can lead to urinary issues and sexual dysfunction. Saw palmetto is widely recognized for its ability to alleviate symptoms associated with BPH, including frequent urination and incomplete bladder emptying.

- By promoting prostate health, saw palmetto may improve urinary function and reduce the pressure on the urinary tract, which can indirectly improve erectile function.

3. **Improved Blood Flow:**

- There is some evidence to suggest that saw palmetto may promote better blood circulation. Healthy blood flow is essential for achieving and maintaining an erection, as erectile dysfunction is often linked to poor circulation.

- Enhanced blood flow to the pelvic region can improve erectile function and overall sexual health.

4. **Anti-Inflammatory Properties:**

o Chronic inflammation can contribute to various health problems, including ED. Saw palmetto has anti-inflammatory properties, which may help reduce inflammation in the prostate and improve overall reproductive health.

o By addressing inflammation, saw palmetto may support the body's natural ability to achieve and maintain erections.

Importance of Saw Palmetto for Erectile Dysfunction

- **Natural Alternative**: Many men seek natural alternatives to pharmaceuticals for managing erectile dysfunction, often due to concerns about side effects or long-term dependence on medications. Saw palmetto offers a more holistic approach to sexual health without the adverse effects associated with some conventional treatments.

- **Long-Term Health Benefits**: In addition to its potential benefits for erectile dysfunction, saw palmetto supports overall prostate health. Maintaining a healthy prostate is crucial for men, especially as they age, to prevent issues like BPH and prostate cancer.

- **Safety Profile**: Saw palmetto is generally well-tolerated and considered safe for most individuals. Unlike some prescription medications, it typically does not produce significant side effects, making it an attractive option for many seeking to improve their sexual health.

How Saw Palmetto Promotes Sexual Health

- **Increased Libido**: By potentially boosting testosterone levels and balancing hormones, saw palmetto may enhance libido, improving sexual desire and performance.
- **Enhanced Erectile Function**: Improved blood flow and prostate health can lead to better erectile function, allowing men to achieve and maintain erections more easily.
- **Reduction in Symptoms of BPH**: Alleviating urinary symptoms associated with BPH can reduce anxiety and stress related to sexual performance, contributing to a healthier sexual experience.

RECIPE AND PREPARATION OF SAW PALMETTO ROOT AT HOME

Saw palmetto can be consumed in various forms, including capsules, extracts, and teas. Here's a simple way to prepare a saw palmetto tea at home using dried saw palmetto berries, which are often available in health food stores or online.

Ingredients:

- 1 tablespoon dried saw palmetto berries
- 2 cups of water
- Optional: Honey or lemon for taste

Preparation:

1. **Crush the Berries**: Start by lightly crushing the dried saw palmetto berries using a mortar and pestle or a rolling pin. This helps release their beneficial compounds.
2. **Boil Water**: In a small saucepan, bring 2 cups of water to a boil.
3. **Steep the Berries**: Once the water is boiling, add the crushed saw palmetto berries to the saucepan. Reduce the heat and let it simmer for about 15-20 minutes.

4. **Strain the Tea**: After steeping, remove the saucepan from heat and strain the mixture using a fine mesh strainer or cheesecloth into a cup or teapot.

5. **Add Flavor (Optional)**: If desired, add honey or lemon to taste. These can enhance the flavor while providing additional health benefits.

6. **Serve and Enjoy**: Drink the tea warm. You can consume this tea 1-2 times a day as part of your routine.

CONCLUSION

In this journey through *The Complete Dr. Barbara's Cure for Erectile Dysfunction*, we've explored a holistic approach to overcoming a condition that affects not only physical health but also emotional well-being and relationships. Erectile dysfunction is a challenge that many men face, but it does not have to define your life. Dr. Barbara's philosophy focuses on treating the body as a whole, addressing the root causes of ED with natural, time-tested remedies that emphasize balance, health, and vitality.

Through dietary changes, lifestyle adjustments, stress management, and natural supplementation—such as the use of saw palmetto and other powerful herbs—we have seen how the body can heal itself when given the right support. By addressing underlying issues like hormonal imbalances, poor circulation, inflammation, and mental health, Dr. Barbara's approach provides a pathway to lasting improvement.

It is important to remember that healing takes time, patience, and persistence. Every positive step you take toward improving your health brings you closer to a more fulfilling and active life. You may not see changes overnight, but with consistent effort, the results can be profound. As you continue applying these natural methods, stay encouraged by the progress you make, even if it comes in small increments.

This book is more than a guide to overcoming erectile dysfunction—it's a roadmap to reclaiming control over your health, self-confidence, and well-being. You now have the tools and knowledge to not only improve your sexual health but also to enhance your overall quality of life.

Believe in your ability to change, to heal, and to thrive. Erectile dysfunction is just one chapter in your life's story—what matters most is how you choose to move forward. With a positive mindset, a healthy lifestyle, and the wisdom shared by Dr. Barbara, you are equipped to take control and live your life to its fullest potential.

Stay committed, stay strong, and remember: your health is your greatest wealth. Here's to a brighter, healthier future!

Made in the USA
Las Vegas, NV
04 November 2024

11100551R00072